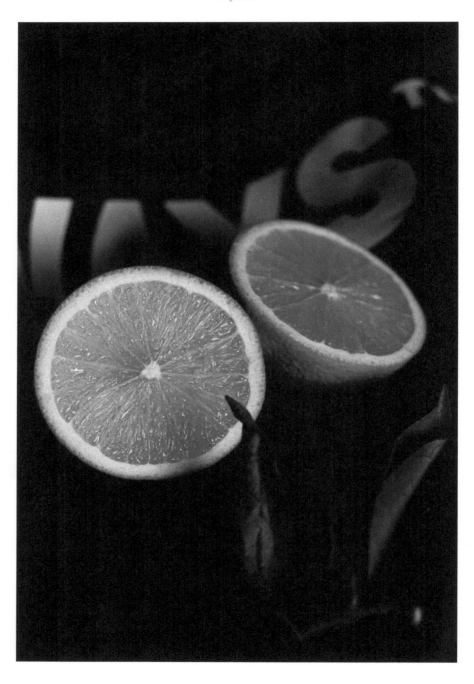

Sirtfood Diet

Lose weight and burn fat with the help of fabulous recipes that activate your SKINNY GENE

Lisa T. Oliver

Contents

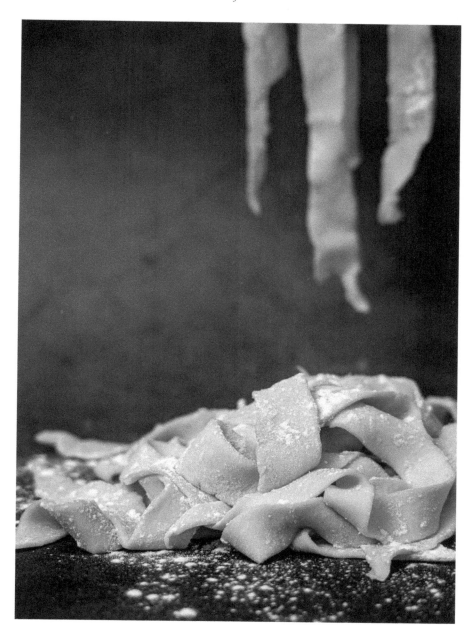

Introduction

What Are Sirtfoods?

Sirtuins refer to a protein class that has been proven to regulate the metabolism of fat and glucose. According to research, sirtuins also have a significant impact on aging, inflammation, and cell death.

By consuming foods rich in sirtuins like cocoa, kale, and parsley, you stimulate your skinny gene pathway and lose fat faster.

About the Sirtfood Diet

The Sirtfood Diet plan considers that some foods activate your "skinny gene" and can make you lose about seven pounds in about a week.Certain foods, such as dark chocolate, kale, and wine, contain polyphenols, a natural chemical that imitates exercise and fasting and affects the body. Other sirtfoods include cinnamon, red onions, and turmeric. These trigger the sirtuins' pathway and start weight loss. There is scientific evidence to support this too. The impact of weight loss is higher in the first week. The Sirtfood Diet mainly consists of plant-based foods that are rich in sirtuins to trigger fat loss. The diet is divided into two phases, which can be repeated continuously.The first phase is three days of living on 1000 calories and four days of 1500 calories with lots of green juices.

The Premise of the Sirtfood Diet The premise of the Sirtfood Diet states that certain foods can mimic the benefits of fasting and caloric restrictions by activating sirtuins, which kare proteins in the body. They range from SIRT1 to SIRT7, switch genes on and off, maintain biological pathways, and protect cells from age-related decline. Although intense calorie restriction and fasting are severe, the Sirtfood Diet inventors developed a plan with a focus on eating plenty of sirtfoods. It's a more natural way to stimulate sirtuin genes in the body, also known as skinny genes. In the process, it improves health and boosts weight loss. If you want to start the Sirtfood Diet, planning is required, and access to the ingredients needed to follow the diet correctly. There are many exciting recipes for the diet, with a variety of ingredients. However, it may often be challenging to get certain ingredients during specific seasons and times of the year. Some of these ingredients include kale and strawberries, for example. It may also be stressful to follow social events when traveling or to care for a young child. The Sirtfood Diet covers various food groups; however, dairy foods aren't included in the plan. Sirtfoods are a new diet discovery. They are rich in nutrients and capable of activating skinny genes in the body, with benefits and downsides alike.

s

The Science of Sirtuins

The Sirtfood diet is very famous due to its scientific benefits and amazing transformations within the body's metabolic capacities. Thousands of people have unlocked incredible and aesthetic physiques by following the Sirtfood diet. These results are not coming from word of mouth or myths attached to basic philosophies of dieting; in fact, the Sirtfood diet has a robust yet growing scientific background. The discovery of the Sirtfood diet was not an accident, but researchers found the necessary components, the polyphenols, in labs and conducted many types of research to conform to the scientific benefits of the Sirtfood diet. The primary lean gene, also known as a sirtuin, on which this dieting style got its name was first found in 1984 and not in humans but in yeasts. Polyphenol is a well-known chemical compound present in the body and acts on an essential lean gene to activate and perform fat-burning blitz inside the human body. To be very specific, Sirtfoods are those which contain high levels of a chemical compound called polyphenol. This compound is not uniformly distributed in Sirtfoods, but every Sirtfood contains specific amounts of polyphenols. The answer is straightforward yet very informative. Polyphenols are the compounds that are present naturally in Sirtfood, and many types of research conducted have confirmed that these foods have the highest impacts when losing extra pounds of fats from the body.

Polyphenols are essential precursors in the fat burning cycle of the body called lipolysis. Free fatty acids in our blood are subjected to digestion and then excretion from the body through an enzyme called lipase. Foods rich in Polyphenols cause much increase in levels of lipase enzyme and thus more fat burning blitz in the body. Polyphenols act on lipase and other fat-burning mediators by activating a particular type of gene in the body called sirtuin. This gene is the most crucial part of the Sirtfood diet because, through this gene activation, polyphenol-rich foods called the Sirtfoods act on extra stored fat in our body and engine a fat-burning cycle in our body to get rid of it. Sirtuin gene is a human gene and present in every human. It is also present in some other animals as well but in modified forms. Interestingly, the very first encounter with the sirtuin gene was in 2002 when a group of researchers found its over-activation associated with particular types of foods given to some animals. Then many studies were conducted on mice to check the efficacy of these foods and the activation of the sirtuin gene in the human body. These trials confirmed that the sirtuin gene is associated with fat loss, and Sirtfoods, which contain the maximum amount of polyphenol, are very important when undergoing a fat loss diet.

It is also fascinating to know that Sirtfoods are not very rare types of food. These foods contain a significant portion of both eastern and western diets as well as in Mediterranean diets. The Sirtfood diet consists of the top twenty foods in the world, which are considered as the basic Sirtfoods. These twenty foods contain the highest amounts of sirtuin-activating polyphenols. The levels of polyphenol are not uniformly distributed in all these foods, and some of them contain higher amounts. Moreover, different types of polyphenols are present in these Sirtfoods, which are associated with special effects on the sirtuin gene. The most important aspect of the Sirtfood diet is that it uses a variety of foods. These twenty Sirtfoods make an essential part of the Sirtfood diet so that the maximum amount of all types of polyphenols is consumed to maximize the fat burning in our body.

CHAPTER 1: The Science Behind the Fat-Burning Benefits of the Sirtfood Diet

The most significant benefit of the Sirtfood diet is its incredible impact on losing fats from the body. Fats are made up of fatty acids that combine to make adipocytes. These adipocytes are clusters of fatty acids, and unlike free fatty acids, adipocytes are not mostly present in the blood. They get accumulated under the skin, in muscles, and on different organs. These adipocytes combine to make adipose tissues, which are full fledge foam-shaped cluster of visible yellowish white-color fat in our body. Adipocytes are the healthiest fat cells to burn, and they must have been broken down into adipocytes and finally in free fatty acids (in reverse order of formation) to get burned from the fat-burning enzymes called the lipase enzyme. These steps are not easy as they seem, and burning extra pounds of fats can be a hard nut to crack. The most challenging step in this cycle is to break adipose tissues in adipocytes. The Sirtfoods contain high levels of polyphenols.

CHAPTER 2: The Sirtfood Diet and Energy Cycle of the Body

The fuel of the body is glucose, which is the most readily available nutrient in the body for energy. The glucose is broken down into energy packets called ATPs, which are produced from the power of cells called mitochondria. These energy packets are utilized to fuel the body while performing actions. High-intensity work such as exercise requires a much more significant amount of energy as compared to typing on a keyboard. The higher the intensity of work, the larger will be the needed number of ATPs. The most significant source of glucose in the body is carbohydrates, which are sugars in simpler forms. A diet rich in low glycemic carbohydrates is essential while performing high-intensity tasks. These carbohydrates are broken down into the purest form of sugar called glucose. This glucose undergoes a series of reactions called glycolysis. In this cycle, the end product is the ATPs that are stored or utilized in response to stress produced in the body. These ATPs are also crucial for fighting against the infections because the higher the level of energy in the body, the greater will be the immune response of the body. All the processes are directly proportional.

The Sirtfood diet is affluent in proteins, good fats, and low glycemic carbohydrates. All these macronutrients are essential for fulfilling the body's essential needs of energy and refueling.

CHAPTER 3: The Sirtfood Diet and Poke Hole Theory

This is by far the most valuable information about the Sirtfood diet. Very brief literature is available about the poke hole theory and its relationship with the Sirtfood diet. When a person undergoes a diet, which comprises of a calorie deficit scenario, our body takes it as a challenge and signals our mitochondria—the powerhouse of the cell to produce ATP, which are the energy packets to supply the body with instant energy. This calorie deficit scenario pokes holes in mitochondria, and thus, specific genes are activated in a cyclic manner to produce a considerable amount of energy in response to these holes in mitochondria. You can say that mitochondria get excited in response to these poked holes. A significant benefit of this cycling production of energy is the utilization of stored fats as a source of energy. When the body is not getting enough from outside sources, it becomes evident that the body must utilize its energy stores either from fat, muscles, or available glucose.

As the energy consumption is higher and calorie intake is higher when someone starts a calorie deficit diet such as the Sirtfood diet, the body acts on cyclic use of its stored fat to mobilize it in blood, and high metabolic rates due to exercise cause consumption and immediate burning of these free fatty acids in the blood. If someone consumes fat mobilizing precursors from the diet, this fat-burning mechanism can speed up too many folds.

CHAPTER 4:

Breakfast

1.   Salmon Burgers

The salmon burger is an exquisite fish second course! A simple, quick, and delicious alternative to the classic meat burger! It is prepared with fresh salmon and aromatic herbs, which give the hamburger an intense aroma and a tasty taste.

Preparation Time: 10 minutes

Cooking Time: 3 minutes

Servings: 4

Ingredients

Quantity for three large or four small burgers

600 gr of salmon slices (the flesh net of scraps will be about 350 gr)

One sprig of fresh dill (optional)

One sprig of fresh parsley

Salt

Two tablespoons of extra virgin olive oil to cook the hamburgers

For the accompanying yogurt sauce:

125 grams of sugar-free white yogurt

some fresh or dry dill (optional)

some fresh parsley

As a side dish or to fill the sandwich (per portion):

around tomato

a handful of valerian or rocket or spinach

a small red onion

extra virgin olive oil

Salt

One soft hamburger sandwich with seeds (only if you want to make a sandwich)

Directions:

First of all, fillet the salmon slices with a sharp knife. Peel off the skin and cut into small pieces, taking care to remove the thorns stuck in the flesh. Don't waste anything; remove only the central bone and outer skin.

Then wash and chop together with a large knife, parsley, and dill.

With the help of a blender with a sharp blade, chop the pieces of salmon; it will take a few seconds to get a delicate and shapely chopping.

Add to the chopped salmon, the flavorings, and salt.

Knead together.

Three large or four small burgers come out from the mixture, so divide the mixture into equal parts.

Form a round, compact ball.

Crush the ball until it is about 1 cm thick and with the palms of your hands, simultaneously shape the edges forming a flattened and shaped circle, until you obtain a hamburger with well-defined sides.

Wash the tomatoes and slice them.

Peel and slice the onion.

Wash the valerian or rocket and dry them. Chop the herbs with a knife and pour them into the yogurt.

2.   Green Omelet

Preparation time: 10 min Cooking time: 5 min Servings: 1

Ingredients:

Two large eggs, at room temperature

1shallot, peeled and chopped

Handful arugula

Three sprigs of parsley, chopped

1tsp extra virgin olive oil

Salt and black pepper

Directions:

Beat the eggs in a small bowl and set aside. Sauté the shallot for 5 minutes with a bit of the oil, on low-medium heat. Pour the eggs into the pans, stirring the mixture for just a second. The eggs on medium heat, and tip the pan just enough to let the loose egg run underneath after about one minute on the burner. Add the greens, herbs, and seasonings to the top side as it is still soft. TIP: You do not even have to flip it, as you can just simmer the egg as is well (being careful not to burn). TIP: Another option is to put it into an oven to broil for 3-5 minutes.

Nutrition: Energy (calories): 99 kcal Protein: 3.67 g Fat: 6.6 g Carbohydrates: 6.81 g

3. Berry Oat Breakfast Cobbler

Preparation time: 40 min

Cooking time: 5 min

Servings: 2

Ingredients:

2 cups of oats/flakes that are ready without cooking

1cup of blackcurrants without the stems

1teaspoon of honey (or ¼ teaspoon of raw sugar)

½ cup of water (add more or less by testing the pan)

1 cup of plain yogurt (or soy or coconut)

Directions:

Boil the berries, honey, and water, and then turn it down on low. Put in a glass container in a refrigerator until it is cold and set (about 30 minutes or more)

When ready to eat, scoop the berries on top of the oats and yogurt. Serve immediately.

Nutrition:

Energy (calories): 802 kcal

Protein: 47.97 g

Fat: 21.42 g Carbohydrates: 176.89 g

4. Granola- The Sirt Way

Preparation time: 30 min

Cooking time: 0 min

Servings: 1

Ingredients:

1 cup buckwheat puffs

1 cup buckwheat flakes (ready to eat type, but not whole buckwheat that needs to be cooked) ½ cup coconut flakes

½ cup Medjool dates, without pits, chopped into smaller, bite-sized pieces

1 cup of cacao nibs or very dark chocolate chips

1/2 cup walnuts, chopped

1 cup strawberries chopped and without stem 1 cup plain Greek, or coconut or soy yogurt.

Directions:

Mix without yogurt and strawberry toppings.

You can store for up to a week. Store in an airtight container. Add toppings (even different berries or different yogurt.

You can even use the berry toppings as you will learn how to make from other recipes.

5.   Summer Berry Smoothie

Preparation time: 30 min

Cooking time: 0 min

Servings: 1

Ingredients

50g (2oz) blueberries

50g (2oz) strawberries

25g (1oz) blackcurrants

25g (1oz) red grapes

1 carrot, peeled

1 orange, peeled

Juice of 1 lime

Directions

Place all of the ingredients into a blender and cover them with water. Blitz until smooth. You can also add some crushed ice and a mint leaf to garnish.

Nutrition:

Energy (calories): 113 kcal

Protein: 1.59 g

Fat: 0.53 g Carbohydrates: 28.94 g

6.   Celery & Ginger Smoothie

Preparation time: 30 min

Cooking time: 0 min

Servings: 1

Ingredients

1stalk of celery

50g (2oz) kale

One apple, cored

50g (2oz) mango, peeled, de-stoned and chopped

2.5cm (1 inch) chunk of fresh ginger root, peeled and chopped

Directions:

Put all the ingredients into a blender with some water and blitz until smooth. Add ice to make your smoothie refreshing.

7.   Orange, Carrot & Kale Smoothie

Preparation time: 30 min

Cooking time: 0 min

Servings: 1

Ingredients

One carrot, peeled

One orange, peeled

One stick of celery

One apple, cored

50g (2oz) kale

½ teaspoon matcha powder

Directions:

Place all of the ingredients into a blender and add in enough water to cover them. Process until smooth, serve, and enjoy.

Nutrition:

Energy (calories): 144 kcal

Protein: 3.18 g Fat: 0.92 g

Carbohydrates: 35.36 g

8.   Creamy Strawberry & Cherry Smoothie

Preparation time: 30 min

Cooking time: 0 min

Servings: 1

Ingredients

100g (3½ oz.) strawberries

75g (3oz) frozen pitted cherries

One tablespoon plain full-fat yogurt

175mls (6fl oz.) unsweetened soya milk

Directions:

Place all of the ingredients into a blender and process until smooth. Serve and enjoy.

Nutrition:

Energy (calories): 108 kcal

Protein: 2.34 g

Fat: 0.63 g

Carbohydrates: 25.53 g

9.   Grape, Celery & Parsley Reviver

Preparation time: 30 min

Cooking time: 0 min

Servings: 1

Ingredients

75g (3oz) red grapes

Three sticks of celery

One avocado, de-stoned and peeled

One tablespoon fresh parsley

½ teaspoon matcha powder

Directions:

Place all of the ingredients into a blender with enough water to cover them and blitz until smooth and creamy. Add crushed ice to make it even more refreshing.

Nutrition:

Energy (calories): 375 kcal

Protein: 4.67 g

Fat: 29.62 g

Carbohydrates: 30.97 g

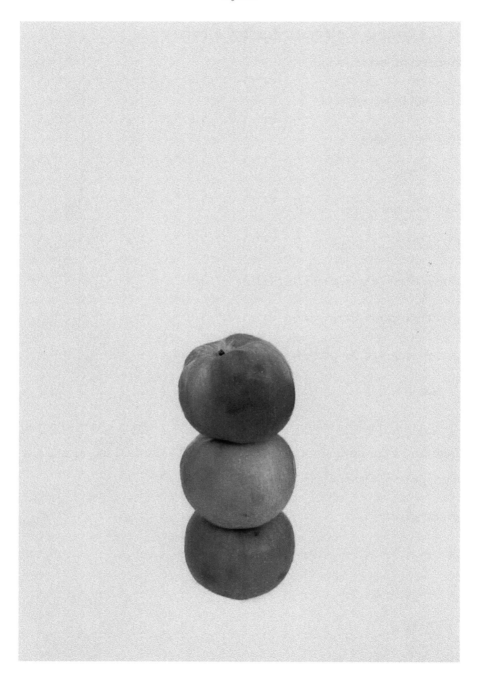

CHAPTER 5:

Lunch

10.   Cilantro Shrimp With Chard, Squash, And Wild Rice

Preparation time: 10 minutes

Cooking time: 15 minutes Servings: 4

Ingredients:

1 Tbsp. of olive oil

Eight large shrimp

2 tsp. of fresh cilantro

One yellow squash, sliced

2 tsp. of fresh lime juice

1 cup of Swiss chard

1/4 cup of dry wild rice blend

Directions:

Sear shrimp in the olive oil over medium heat for 3-4 minutes, seasoning with lime juice and cilantro.

Steam chard and squash for 5-7 minutes, and cook rice according to the package directions.

Nutrition:

Energy (calories): 197 kcal

Protein: 3.35 g

Fat: 14.86 g

Carbohydrates: 13.89 g

11.   Lemon Chicken With Gazpacho

Preparation time: 10 minutes

Cooking time: 35 minutes

Servings: 4

Ingredients (chicken):

1 Tbsp. of olive oil

3 1/2 oz. of chicken breast

1 tsp. of fresh rosemary

1/2 lemon, sliced

Ingredients (gazpacho):

Three cloves of garlic, minced

1 cup of stewed tomatoes

1/2 cup of onion, chopped

1/4 cup of cucumber, chopped

1 Tbsp. of white wine vinegar

1/4 cup of green pepper, chopped

Directions:

Coat chicken with some olive oil. Cover with rosemary and lemon slices, and bake at 350°F for about 25 to 30 minutes.

Combine gazpacho ingredients in a blender and serve at room temperature with chicken.

Nutrition:

nergy (calories): 362 kcal

Protein: 23.33 g

Fat: 23.22 g

Carbohydrates: 15.81 g

12. Zesty Tofu And Quinoa

Preparation time: 20 minutes

Cooking time: 0 minutes

Servings: 4

Ingredients:

2 oz. of extra-firm tofu, cubed

1 cup of cooked quinoa

3 Tbsp. of diced red pepper

1 tsp. of cilantro

2 Tbsp. of diced avocado

3 Tbsp. of chopped green pepper

2 tsp. of fresh lime juice

Directions:

Combine all ingredients.

Nutrition:

Energy (calories): 982 kcal

Protein: 24.81 g

Fat: 66.15 g

Carbohydrates: 90.14 g

13.   Confetti Pesto Pasta

Preparation time: 10 minutes

Cooking time: 25 minutes

Servings: 4

Ingredients:

1/3 cup of cooked green beans

1/4 pint of cherry tomatoes

1/3 cup of diced chicken breast

1/4 tsp. of each salt and pepper

1 cup of cooked linguine

1/4 cup of pesto sauce

1/4 cup of shredded Parmesan

Directions:

Combine tomatoes, diced chicken breast, cooked green beans, pesto sauce, pepper, and salt in a bowl. Add cooked linguine. Garnish with shredded Parmesan.

Nutrition:

Energy (calories): 865 kcal

Protein: 35.75 g

Fat: 44.25 g Carbohydrates: 88.94 g

14.   Asian Turkey Lettuce Cups

Preparation time: 10 minutes

Cooking time: 15 minutes

Servings: 4

Ingredients (turkey):

1/2 cup of white mushrooms, chopped

4 oz. of lean ground turkey

1/4 cup of shelled and cooked edamame

1 tsp. of minced garlic

2 Tbsp. of sliced scallion

2 Boston lettuce leaves

Ingredients (sauce):

1 tsp. of low-sodium soy sauce

1/2 Tbsp. of hoisin sauce

1/2 tsp. of rice vinegar

Ingredients (slaw):

1/2 cup of shredded green cabbage and red cabbage

1/4 cup of grated carrot

1/4 cup of sliced jicama

1/2 tsp. of rice vinegar

1 tsp. of olive oil

Directions:

In the nonstick skillet coated with cooking spray, sauté the first three ingredients for 5 minutes.

Add edamame, scoop mix with lettuce, top with scallion, and then wrap it up.

Drizzle together with the sauce, and serve slaw on the side.

Nutrition:

Energy (calories): 334 kcal

Protein: 29.14 g

Fat: 16.63 g

Carbohydrates: 19.83 g

15.   Pork With Roasted Vegetables

Preparation time: 10 minutes

Cooking time: 25 minutes

Servings: 4

Ingredients:

1 cup of baked cubed butternut squash

3 oz. of pork tenderloin

1 tsp. of black pepper

2 cups of brussels sprouts cooked in 1 tab of olive oil

1/2 tsp. of salt

Directions:

Roast pork tenderloin at 375°F, and serve with vegetables.

Nutrition:

Energy (calories): 323 kcal

Protein: 32.37 g

Fat: 4.83 g

Carbohydrates: 45.51 g

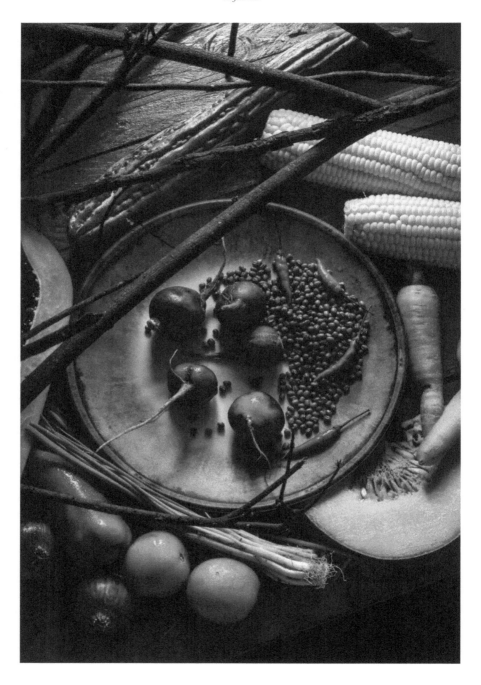

CHAPTER 6:

Dinner

16.   Miso-Marinated Prepared Cod

Preparation Time: 40 min.

Cooking Time: 10 minutes

Servings: 2

Ingredients:

20g miso

1tbsp mirin

1tbsp additional virgin olive oil

200g skinless cod filet

20g red onion, cut

40g celery, cut

One clove garlic, finely hacked

1 10,000 foot bean stew, finely cleaved

1tsp new ginger, finely slashed

60g green beans

50g kale, generally hacked

30g buckwheat

1tsp ground turmeric

1tsp sesame seeds

5g parsley, commonly hacked

1tbsp tamari or soy sauce

Directions:

Heat the stove to 220°C/200°C fan/gas mark 7.

Mix the miso, mirin, and 1tsp oil, rub into the cod and marinate for 30 minutes. Move on to a heating plate and cook for 10 minutes.

Meanwhile, heat an enormous skillet with the rest of the oil. Include the onion and sautéed food for a couple of moments, including the celery, garlic, stew, ginger, green beans, and kale. Fry until the kale is delicate and cooked through, adding a little water to soften the kale if required.

Cook the buckwheat according to pack directions with the turmeric. Include the sesame seeds, parsley, and tamari or soy sauce

To the pan-fried food and present with the greens and fish.

Nutrition:Energy (calories): 474 kcal Protein: 55.59 g Fat: 15.61 g Carbohydrates: 29.24 g

17. Sirt Super Plate Of Mixed Greens

Preparation Time: 20 min.

Cooking Time: 10 minutes

Servings: 2

Ingredients:

50g rocket

50g chicory leaves

100g smoked salmon cuts

80g avocado, stripped, stoned, and cut

40g celery, cut

20g red onion, cut

15g pecans, hacked

1tbsp tricks

One huge Medjool date, hollowed and slashed

1tbsp additional virgin olive oil

Juice 1/2 lemon

10g parsley, cleaved

10g lovage or celery leaves, cleaved

Mix every one of the fixings and serve.

Chargrilled meat

100g potatoes, stripped and diced into 2cm 3D shapes

1tbsp additional virgin olive oil

5g parsley, finely cleaved

50g red onion, cut into rings

50g kale, cleaved

One clove garlic, finely cleaved

120-150g 3.5cm-thick meat filet

steak or 2cm-thick sirloin steak

40ml red wine

150ml meat stock

1tsp tomato purée

1tsp cornflour broke down in 1tbsp water

Directions:

Heat the stove to 220°C/200°C fan/gas mark 7.

Place the potatoes in a pan of bubbling water, bring to the bubble and cook for 4-5 minutes, then channel. Spot in a simmering tin with 1tsp oil and cook for 35-45 minutes, turning at regular intervals. Expel from the stove, sprinkle with the cleaved parsley and blend well.

Fry the onion in 1tsp oil over medium warmth until delicate and caramelized. Keep warm.

Steam the kale for 2-3 minutes, then channel. Fry the garlic delicately in 1/2tsp oil for one moment until delicate. Include the kale and fry for a further 1-2 minutes, until tender. Keep warm. Heat an ovenproof griddle until smoking. Coat the meat in 1/2tsp oil and fry according to how you like it done. Expel from the dish and put aside to rest. Add the wine to the hot skillet to raise any meat buildup. Air pocket to decrease the wine considerably until it's syrupy with a concentrated flavor.

Add the stock and tomato purée to the steak container and bring to the bubble, then add the cornflour glue to thicken the sauce a little at once until you have the ideal consistency. Mix in any juice from the refreshed steak and present with the potatoes, kale, onion rings, and red wine sauce.

18.   Prepared Chicken Bosom

Preparation Time: 10 min.

Cooking Time: 30 minutes

Servings: 2

Ingredients:

For the pesto

15g parsley

15g pecans

15g Parmesan

1tbsp additional virgin olive oil

Juice 1/2 lemon

For the chicken

150g skinless chicken bosom

20g red onions, finely cut

1tsp red wine vinegar

35g rocket

100g cherry tomatoes, split

1tsp balsamic vinegar

Directions:

Heat the stove to 220°C/200°C fan/gas mark 7.

To make the pesto, mix the parsley, pecans, Parmesan, olive oil, a large portion of the lemon juice, and 1 tbsp water in a nourishment processor until you have

Smooth glue. Step by step, include more water until you have your favored consistency.

Marinate chicken bosom in 1 tbsp of the pesto and the rest of the lemon squeeze in the more relaxed for 30 minutes, or more if conceivable.

In an ovenproof griddle over medium-high warmth, fry the chicken in its marinade for one moment on either side, then exchange the skillet to the stove and cook for 8 minutes, or until cooked through.

Marinate the onions in the red wine vinegar for 5-10 minutes, then channel off the fluid.

When the chicken is cooked, expel it from the stove, spoon over 1 tbsp pesto, and let the chicken's warmth dissolve the pesto. Spread with foil and leave to rest for 5 minutes before serving.

Combine the rocket, tomatoes, and onion and shower over the balsamic. Present with the chicken, spooning throughout the remainder of the pesto.

19. Loaded Spaghetti

Preparation time: 20minutes

Cooking time: 0 minutes

Servings: 4

Ingredients:

1/2 cup of sliced red onion

1 cup of sliced bell pepper

1 tsp. of olive oil

2/3 cup of cooked edamame

1 cup of cooked whole-wheat spaghetti

Directions:

Put onions and sauté peppers in oil until the onions are translucent. Toss with edamame and pasta.

Nutrition: Energy (calories): 616 kcal Protein: 28.69 g Fat: 13.05 g Carbohydrates: 106.32 g

20. Mediterranean Shrimp

Preparation time: 10 minutes

Cooking time: 25 minutes Servings: 4

Ingredients:

1 lb. of large shrimp — 40 - 50 per pound peeled, deveined shrimp, tails on or off (frozen or fresh and thawed)

½ tsp. of ground black pepper — divided

¾ tsp. of kosher salt — divided

2 Tbsp. of extra virgin olive oil

Two cloves of garlic — minced (about 2 tsp.)

One small red onion — chopped

One 14.5-oz can of fire-roasted diced tomatoes in their juices

1 tsp. of dried oregano

1 tsp. of honey

¼ tsp. of red pepper flakes

1 tsp. of red wine vinegar

½ c. of pitted Kalamata olives

One 14-oz can of artichoke hearts — drained & quartered

¾ c. of crumbled feta cheese

2 Tbsp. of fresh lemon juice — from ½ medium lemon

2 Tbsp. of chopped fresh parsley

For serving: rice — whole wheat couscous, pasta (optional), crusty bread

Directions:

Place rack at the middle of your oven and preheat the oven to 400 degrees F. Dry the shrimp, put in a mixing bowl, and sprinkle with 1/2 tsp. of salt and 1/4 tsp. of black pepper. Toss to coat, and then set aside.

Heat the oil (olive) in a large, ovenproof skillet over medium heat. Add the onion and sprinkle with the remaining 1/4 teaspoon of salt and 1/4 teaspoon of black pepper. Cook, occasionally stirring, until cooled, for about 5 minutes. Reduce heat as needed to soften the onion, but not brown. Add the garlic and cook until fragrant, about 30 seconds.Substitute the onion, oregano, and red pepper flakes. Reduce heat to medium-low and simmer gently for 10 minutes. Stir in the vinegar of red wine and honey. Remove it from the heat.Lay the artichokes and olives over the top, spread tomatoes, and then place the shrimp over the top in a single layer. Sprinkle it with the feta.Bake for 10 - 12 minutes until the tomatoes burst, the cheese is lightly browned, and the shrimp is cooked through. Squeeze some juice of the lemon over the top and scatter with the parsley. Enjoy the hot one.

Nutrition: 24 g fat, 445 calories, 38 g protein, 9 g sugars, 17 g carb, 3 g fiber.

CHAPTER 7:

Mains

21.　Sirtfood Pizza

Preparation Time: 10 minutes.

Cooking Time: 60minutes

Servings: 6

Ingredients:

7g dry yeast

1 tsp. brown sugar

300ml water

200g buckwheat flour

200g wheat flour for pasta

1 tbsp. olive oil

Directions:

Dissolve dry yeast and sugar in water and leave covered for 15 minutes. Then mix the flours. Add the yeast water and oil and make a dough.

Preheat oven to 425 °. Then knead the dough well again and form two pizzas, each 30 cm in diameter, with a rolling pin on a floured work surface. Or you can develop a thin pizza that fits on a whole baking sheet.

Spread the pizza dough on a baking tray lined with baking paper

For the sauce

1/2 red onion, finely chopped

One clove garlic, finely chopped

1 tsp. olive oil

1 tsp. oregano, dried

2 tbsps. red wine

One can of strained tomatoes (400ml)

1 pinch brown sugar

5g basil leaves

Directions:

Fry the garlic, onion, and sugar with olive oil, add the wine and oregano, and cook briefly. Then add the tomatoes and cook on low heat for 30 minutes. Then set aside and add the fresh basil leaves.

Pizza topping and baking

Spread the desired amount of tomato sauce on the dough - leave the edges as free as possible, do not spread too thickly.

Then add the desired ingredients, for example

Sliced red onion and grilled eggplant

Goat cheese and cherry tomatoes

Chicken breast (grilled), red onions, and olives

Kale, chorizo, and red onions

Then bake for about 12 minutes and, if desired, sprinkle with rocket, pepper, and chili flakes.

22.   Red Coleslaw

Preparation Time: 10 minutes.

Cooking Time: 10 minutes

Servings: 4

Ingredients:

1 2/3 lbs. red cabbage

2 tbsps. ground caraway seeds

1 tbsp. whole grain mustard

1 1/4 c. mayonnaise, low fat, low sodium

Salt and black pepper

Directions:

Cut the red cabbage into small slices.

Take a large-sized bowl and add all the ingredients alongside cabbage. Mix well, season with salt and pepper. Serve and enjoy!

Nutrition:

80Calories Total Fat 5g

Total Carbohydrate 7g

Protein 1g

23.   Amazing Garlic Aioli

Preparation Time: 5minutes.

Cooking Time: 5 minutes

Servings: 4

Ingredients:

½ c. mayonnaise, low fat and low sodium

Two garlic cloves, minced

Juice of 1 lemon

1 tbsp. fresh-flat leaf Italian parsley, chopped

1 tsp. chives, chopped

Salt and pepper to taste

Directions:

Add mayonnaise, garlic, parsley, lemon juice, chives, and season with salt and pepper.

Blend until combined well.Pour into refrigerator and chill for 30 minutes.

Serve and use as needed!

Nutrition: Calories80 Total Fat 9g Total Carbohydrate 1g Protein 0g

24.   Herbed Tomato And Cheese Salad

Preparation Time: 10 minutes.

Cooking Time: 10 minutes Servings: 4

Ingredients:

1 tsp. Basil, ground

1 tsp. Black pepper

8 Tomatoes sliced in half

1 tsp. Paprika, ground

2 tbsps. Extra virgin olive oil

2 tbsps. Parsley chopped

8 Mozzarella cheese slices

4 tbsps. Lemon juice

Directions:

Drizzle the lemon juice on the inside parts of the sliced tomatoes and then sprinkles them with basil and black pepper.Set two tomato halves on each of four serving plates. Place one slice of cheese on each tomato half and then sprinkle on the paprika and the parsley.Sprinkle the olive oil over the tomatoes and serve.

Nutrition:Calories269 Total Fat 10.3g Sodium 730mg Protein 11.2g

CHAPTER 8:

Meat

25. Turkey With Sirtfood Vegetables

This recipe is highly adjustable, and it's based on combining turkey as the main dish with healthy side-dishes made of vegetables. It's effortless and convenient, as meats go great with all Sirt spices and vegetables. With that in mind, feel free to adjust or replace any ingredient in this recipe with an equal amount of the elements you prefer or like better.

Preparation Time: 10 min.

Cooking Time: 30 minutes

Servings: 2

Ingredients:

Lean turkey meat, 150 g

One finely chopped garlic clove

One finely chopped red onion

One finely chopped bird's eye chili/replace with chopped red bell paprika, or ½ squeezed citrus fruit if you don't like spicy foods

1 tsp. of finely chopped ginger

Extra virgin olive oil, 2 tbsp.

Ground turmeric 1 tbsp.

½ cup of dried tomatoes

Parsley, 10 g

Sage, dried, 1 tsp.

½ juiced lime or lemon

Capers 1 tbsp.

Directions:

Chop the cauliflower. Fry with chopped ginger, chili, red onion, and garlic in 1 tbsp. Olive oil until they're soft. Add cauliflower and turmeric, and cook for a couple of minutes until the cauliflower becomes soft. Once the dish is done, add dried tomatoes and parsley.

Coat your turkey in a thin layer of olive oil and sage. Fry for about five minutes, and then add the capers and lime juice to the mix. Add half a cup of water and bring to a boil.

CHAPTER 9:

Sides

26.   Avocado Mint Soup

Preparation Time: 10 Minutes

Cooking Time: 10 Minutes

Servings: 2

Ingredients:

One medium avocado, peeled, pitted, and cut into pieces

1 cup of coconut milk

Two romaine lettuce leaves

20 fresh mint leaves

1 tbsp. fresh lime juice

1/8 tsp. salt

Directions:

Combine all materials into the blender.

The soup should be thick, not as a puree. Wait and blend until it is smooth.

Pour into the serving bowls and place in the refrigerator for 10 minutes.

Stir well and serve chilled.

Nutrition: Calories 268 Fat 25.6 G Carbohydrates 10.2 G Sugar 0.6 G Protein 2.7 G Cholesterol 0 mg

27.   Cucumber Edamame Salad

Preparation Time: 5 Minutes

Cooking Time: 8 Minutes

Servings: 2

Ingredients:

3 tbsp. Avocado oil

1 cup cucumber, sliced into thin rounds

½ cup fresh sugar snap peas cut up or whole

½ cup fresh edamame

¼ cup radish, sliced

One large avocado, peeled, pitted, sliced

One nori sheet crumbled

2 tsp. Roasted sesame seeds

1 tsp. Salt

Directions:

Make a medium-sized pot filled halfway with water to a boil over medium-high heat.

Add the sugar snaps and cook them for about 2 minutes.

Remove the pot off the heat, drain the excess water, transfer the sugar snaps to a medium-sized bowl, and set aside

Fill the pot with water again, add the teaspoon of salt and bring to a boil over medium-high heat.

Add the edamame to the pot and let them cook for about 6 minutes.

Take the pot off the heat, drain the excess water, transfer the soybeans to the bowl with sugar snaps, and cool down for about 5 minutes.

Combine all ingredients, except for the nori crumbs and roasted sesame seeds, in a medium-sized bowl.

Delicately stir, using a spoon, until all ingredients are evenly coated in oil.

Top the salad along with the nori crumbs and roasted sesame seeds.

Shift the bowl to the fridge and allow the salad to cool for at least 30 minutes.

Serve chilled and enjoy!

Nutrition: Calories 409 Carbohydrates 7.1 g Fats 38.25 g Protein 7.6 g

CHAPTER 10:

Seafood

28. Seafood Paella

Preparation time: 10 minutes

Cooking time: 25 minutes

Servings: 4

Ingredients:

620 g riced cauliflower (1 extra-large cauliflower)

1/2 onion

Three garlic cloves

(300g) skinless chicken thighs

130 g about eight scallops

170 g clams weight with the shell/mussels

350 g about 17 shrimps Argentinian Red

Two pinches saffron threads/1/2 tsp. turmeric powder

1 tsp. turmeric powder

100 g green beans

1/2 tsp. thyme

1 1/4 tsp. Himalayan salt

1 1/4 tsp. black pepper

1/2 cup diced tomato can (120ml)

1/2 cup chicken stock

4 tbsp. extra virgin olive oil

2 tbsp. chopped parsley

Directions:

Chop onion. Mince the garlic cloves. Remove the stems off the green beans.

Cut the chicken thighs into bite-size pieces.

Remove the veins from the shrimps. Keep their tails.

In a small bowl, add chicken with 1 tsp. of turmeric powder, minced garlic, thyme, and 1/4 tsp. of salt and pepper. Mix and marinate for a few minutes.

Add 2 tbsp. Of olive oil, diced onion, and riced cauliflower in a wok. Cook for a couple of minutes.

Cook chicken with remaining olive oil in a separate pan. Cook the chicken for 1-2 minutes and finally mix it in with the cauliflower.

Add the threads of saffron, and the diced tomato can, the chicken bouillon, 1 tsp. of salt and pepper, and cover with shrimps, scallops, clams, and green beans.

Cover with steam; cook the seafood for 5 minutes, or until all the clams open.

Uncover, remove the seafood and green beans and place them on the side in a small bowl, allowing the liquid to cook for 3-4 minutes while mixing the chicken and cauliflower rice.

When all the liquid is evaporated, add the seafood back to the saucepan and place it carefully. Add the chopped parsley overall, and turn off the heat

29.   Creamy Fish Casserole

Preparation time: 10 minutes

Cooking time: 20minutes

Servings: 4

Ingredients:

2 tbsp. olive oil

1 lb. broccoli

Six scallions

2 tbsp. small capers

1 oz. butter, for greasing the casserole dish

1½ lbs. white fish, in serving-sized pieces

1¼ cups heavy whipping cream

1 tbsp. Dijon mustard

1 tsp. Salt

¼ tsp. ground black pepper

1 tbsp. dried parsley

3 oz. butter

For Serving

5 oz. leafy greens

Directions:

Let the temperature of the oven set to (200°C).

Cut the broccoli into small florets, including the stem.

On medium-high, fry broccoli for 5 minutes until soft and golden. Add salt and pepper.

Add scallions and capers. Continue to fry for another 2 minutes. Put the vegetables in an oiled baking tray.

Add the fish to the vegetables.

Mix the whipping cream, parsley, and mustard.

Add it over the fish and vegetables.

Add butter slices.

Bake for 20 minutes in the oven until the fish is cooked and flakes easily. Serve as is or with a luscious green salad.

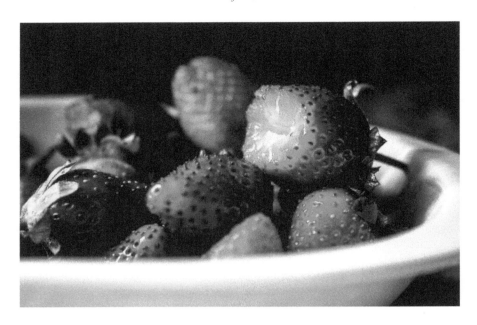

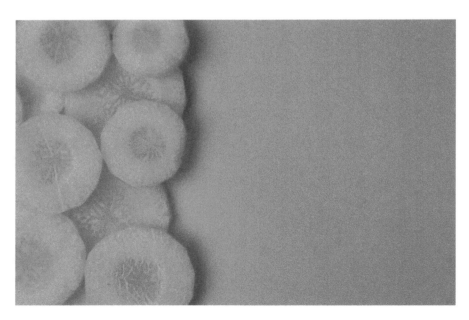

CHAPTER 11:

Poultry

30.   Chicken Salad

Preparation time: 10 minutes

Cooking time: 25 minutes

Servings: 4

Ingredients

For the Buffalo chicken salad:

Two chicken breasts (225 g) peeled, boned, cut in half

Two tablespoons of hot cayenne pepper sauce (or another type of hot sauce), plus an addition depending on taste

Two tablespoons of olive oil

Two hearts of romaine lettuce, cut into 2 cm strips

Four celery stalks, finely sliced

Two carrots, roughly grated

Two fresh onions, only the green part, sliced

125 ml of blue cheese dressing, recipe to follow

For the seasoning of blue cheese

Two tablespoons mayonnaise

70 ml of partially skimmed buttermilk

70 ml low-fat white yogurt

One tablespoon of wine vinegar

½ teaspoon of sugar

35 g of chopped blue cheese

Salt and freshly ground black pepper

Directions:

For the Buffalo chicken salad:

Preheat the grid.

Place the chicken between 2 sheets of baking paper and beat it with a meat tenderizer so that it is about 2 cm thick, then cut the chicken sideways, creating 1 cm strips.

In a large bowl, add the hot sauce and oil, add the chicken and turn it over until it is well soaked. Place the chicken on a baking tray and grill until well cooked, about 4-6 minutes, turning it once.

In a large bowl, add the lettuce, celery, grated carrots, and fresh onions. Add the seasoning of blue cheese. Distribute the vegetables into four plates and arrange the chicken on each of the dishes. Serve with hot sauce on the side.

For the blue cheese dressing:

Cover a small bowl with absorbent paper folded in four. Spread the yogurt on the paper and put it in the fridge for 20 minutes to drain and firm it.

In a medium bowl, beat the buttermilk and frozen yogurt with mayonnaise until well blended. Add the vinegar and sugar and keep beating until well blended. Add the blue cheese and season with salt and pepper to taste.

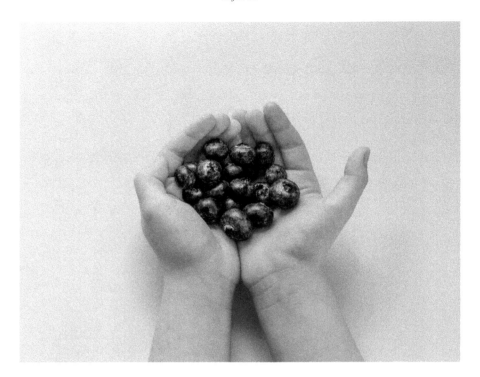

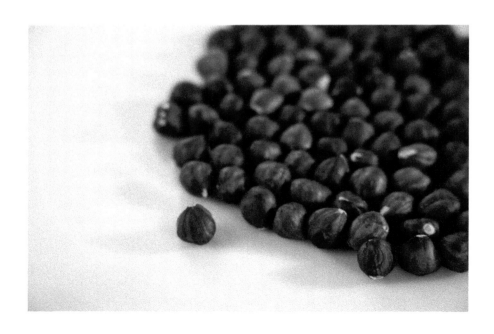

CHAPTER 12:

Vegetable

31. Fermented Pumpkin Vegetables

Preparation Time: 15 min.

Cooking Time: 0 minute

Servings: 1

Ingredients:

One little pumpkin

Spices of your decision, for example, B. mustard seeds and curry

1-2 tablespoons of salt

Directions:

Cut the pumpkin into the littlest potential cuts or pieces.

Mix the cut pumpkin with salt and flavors. Stir the blend appropriately, applying some weight until fluid departures. On the off chance that it doesn't, include some spring water. Now the vegetables, including the subsequent brackish water, are layered in an artistic pot. Continuously leave some space in the compartment and don't top it off to the top. Spread the vegetables with a plate, which you likewise burden. This assists with crushing out the overabundance of air. Set the container aside for seven days at room temperature. You can likewise stand by longer and strengthen the taste. Your tolerance has paid off; you would now be able to eat your first self-aged vegetables.

32. Parsley Butter Asparagus

Preparation Time: 10 minutes

Cooking time: 15 minutes

Servings: 4

Ingredients:

9 oz. asparagus

¼ cup fresh parsley, chopped

Two tablespoons butter

One teaspoon ground paprika

½ teaspoon salt

1 cup water for cooking

Directions:

Pour water into the pan and bring it to a boil. Meanwhile, trim the asparagus and cut it into halves. Put the prepared asparagus in the boiling water and boil for 5 minutes. Then drain water and chill asparagus in the ice water. Toss butter in the saucepan. Melt it. Add chilled asparagus and stir gently. When the asparagus is coated in the butter, sprinkle it with ground paprika and salt.

Close the lid and cook the side dish for 10 minutes over medium-low heat.

Nutrition: calories 67, fat 5.9, fiber 1.7, carbs 3, protein 1.7

33. Baked Bell Peppers With Oil Dressing

Preparation Time: 10 minutes

Cooking time: 10 minutes

Servings: 2

Ingredients:

8 oz. green bell peppers (appx. four bell peppers)

Four tablespoons olive oil ½ teaspoon minced garlic

¼ teaspoon chili flakes ½ teaspoon dried cilantro

½ teaspoon paprika ½ teaspoon salt

Directions:

Pierce the bell peppers with the help of a knife and place them in the tray.

Bake the peppers for 10 minutes at 385F. Flip the peppers onto another side after 5 minutes of cooking. Meanwhile, make oil dressing: whisk together olive oil, minced garlic, chili flakes, dried cilantro, paprika, and salt. When the bell peppers are baked, remove them from the oven and chill a little. Then peel the peppers and clean from the seeds.

Sprinkle the bell peppers with the oil dressing and mix up gently.

Nutrition: calories 267, fat 28.3, fiber 2.2, carbs 6.1 protein 1.2

CHAPTER 13:

Soup, Curries and Stews

34.   Soup The Grandmother's Way

Preparation Time: 10 minutes

Cooking Time: 60 minutes

Servings: 4

Ingredients:

1½ kg chicken (1 chicken)

Three onions

Two inlet leaves

12 dark peppercorns

Salt

300 g celeriac (0.5 celeriac)

400 g giant carrots (3 enormous carrots)

150 g little leek (1 small leek)

150 g parsnips (2 parsnips)

150 g parsley root (3 parsley roots)

200 g Hokkaido pumpkin (1 piece)

175 g entire grain vermicelli

Two stems lovage

Directions:

Wash the chicken, put it in a pot, and convey to the bubble, secured with 3 l of water.

Remove the foam rising upwards with a froth trowel.

Within the interim, unpeel the onions down the center and meal them enthusiastically during a container on the cut surfaces over high warmth without fat.

Add onions with narrows leaves, peppercorns, and somewhat salt to the skimmed stock, stew for quarter-hour on low warmth, flipping if fundamental.

Peel and clean 50% of the celery and carrots. Clean and wash half the leek. Generally, dice everything.

Put the readied vegetables within the pot and cook over medium warmth for 1/2 hours.

Remaining celery, remaining carrots, cleaning, and stripping the parsnips and parsley roots. Clean and wash the pumpkin and remaining leek. Cut everything into 2 cm 3D shapes or cuts.

Take the back off of the soup. Expel the skin and segregate the meat from the bones.

Cut the meat into 2 cm 3D squares and put it in a safe spot.

Pour the soup through a sifter into a subsequent pot; cook the diced vegetables in it over medium warmth for 10-15 minutes. Heat the pasta in salted water, channel, hold quickly under running, cold water (alarm), and increase the soup with the meat and heat. Wash lovage, shake dry, and pluck the leaves. Serve the soup sprinkled with the leaves.

35.   Caldo Verde - Portuguese Kale Soup

Ingredients:

½ kg of potatoes or only a few medium bits of

About 2-3 bunches of hacked kale (without thick stalks)

Less than 1 liter of vegetable stock

1white onion One clove of garlic

One tablespoon of vegetable oil

1-2 tsp. smoked peppers (for soup and serving)

Salt, pepper Toppings:

smoked tempeh, seared tofu, firm roll (discretionary)

Directions:

Fry finely cleaved onion in vegetable oil and ground garlic on a more significant. dd the recently stripped and diced potatoes and fry for around 10 minutes alongside the onion. Then pour the whole stock and cook until the potatoes are delicate. Pull out an outsized portion of the potatoes during a steady progression, forget during a bowl for a few times, and blend the soup during a pot in with a hand blender. At that time, including the rest of the potatoes and hacked kale pieces. Cook for a few moments until the kale relaxes and features light green shading.

Season the soup with liberal pepper and salt and smoked paprika. Serve with seared tempeh or tofu and eat with a fresh roll.

36. Swabian Stew

Preparation Time: 10 minutes

Cooking Time: 45 minutes

Servings: 4

Ingredients:

Two onions

600 g bubbled hamburger

Salt

250 g carrots (2 carrots)

275 g potatoes

200 g celeriac (1 piece)

One stick leek

200 g wholegrain spaetzle

Pepper

2 stems parsley

Directions:

Halve onions and dish with the chop surfaces looking down during a hot skillet without including fat over medium warmth.

Rinse the meat cold. A spot during a pot with the onions and 1 tsp. Salt and spread with approx. 2 l cold water.

Bring back the bubble and evacuate the rising dim froth with the trowel. Decrease the heat and stew the meat over medium warmth for an aggregate of two hours.

Within the interim, wash and strip carrots, potatoes, and celery. Cut everything into 1 cm solid shapes. Put potatoes in chilly water so that they don't change shading.

Halve the leek lengthways and wash under running water. Dig 1 cm wide rings.

Remove the onions from the stock 35 minutes before the cooking time, including the celery and carrots. Further quarter-hour, including the depleted potato shapes and, therefore, the leek.

Cook the spaetzle in bubbling salted water as indicated by the bundle directions. Deplete and extinguish cold.

At the cooking time, remove the meat from the stock and dig reduced down 3D squares.

Add the meat solid shapes with the spaetzle to the stock and heat— season with salt and pepper. Wash the parsley, shake dry, cleave and sprinkle with the stew.

CHAPTER 14:

Snacks & Desserts

37.   Parsley Hummus

Preparation time: 10 minutes

Cooking time: 7 minutes

Servings: 6

Ingredients:

Chickpeas drained and rinsed – 15 ounces

Curly parsley stems removed – 1 cup

Sea salt – .5 teaspoon

Soy milk, unsweetened - .5 cup

Extra virgin olive oil – 3 teaspoons

Lime juice – 1 tablespoon

Red pepper flakes -...5 teaspoons

Black pepper, ground - .25 teaspoon

Pine nuts – 2 tablespoons

Sesame seeds, toasted – 2 tablespoons

Directions:

In the food processor, pulse the parsley and toasted sesame seeds until it forms a fine powdery texture. Drizzle in the extra virgin olive oil while you continue to beat until it is smooth.

Add the chickpeas, lime juice, and seasonings to the food processor and pulse while slowly adding in the soy milk. Continue to pulse the parsley hummus until it is smooth and creamy.

Adjust the seasonings to your preference and then serve or refrigerate the hummus.

Nutrition:

Energy (calories): 210 kcal

Protein: 6.65 g

Fat: 16.19 g

Carbohydrates: 12.63g

38.   Edamame Hummus

Preparation time: 8 minutes

Cooking time: 7 minutes

Servings: 10

Ingredients:

Edamame, cooked and shelled – 2 cups

Sea salt – 1 teaspoon

Extra virgin olive oil – 1 tablespoon

Tahini paste - .25 cup

Lemon juice - .25 cup

Garlic, minced – 3 cloves

Black pepper, ground - .25 teaspoon

Directions:

Add the cooked edamame and remaining ingredients to a blender or food processor and mix on high until it forms a creamy and completely smooth mixture. Taste it and adjust the seasonings to your preference.

Serve the hummus immediately with your favorite vegetables or store it in the fridge.

Nutrition: Energy (calories): 589 kcal Protein: 37.16 g Fat: 30.44g Carbohydrates: 50.34 g

39.   Edamame Guacamole

Preparation time: 10 minutes

Cooking time: 7 minutes

Servings: 6

Ingredients:

Edamame, cooked and shelled – 1 cup

Avocado pitted and halved – 1

Red onion, diced - .5 cup

Cilantro, chopped - .25 cup

Jalapeno, minced – 1

Garlic, minced – 2 cloves

Lime juice – 2 tablespoons

Water – 3 tablespoons

Lime zest - .5 teaspoon

Roma tomato, diced – 2

Cumin - .125 teaspoon

Sea salt - .5 teaspoon

The Directions:

Into a blender or food processor, add all of the ingredients, except for the diced tomato, onion, and jalapeno. Blend the tomato mixture on high speed until it is smooth and creamy, ensuring that the edamame has been thoroughly blended. Adjust the seasoning to your preference, and then transfer the guacamole to a serving bowl. Stir in the tomato, onion, and jalapeno. Place the bowl in the fridge, allowing it to chill for at least thirty minutes before serving.

Nutrition:

Energy (calories): 584 kcal

Protein: 23.94 g Fat: 38.13 g

Carbohydrates: 49.58 g

40. Eggplant Fries With Fresh Aioli

These fries are delicious with fresh aioli, but feel free to experiment with serving them with various dips and sauces. You might find that you love these fries so much that you aren't content to have them as only a snack but also as a side dish.

Preparation time: 10 minutes

Cooking time: 25 minutes

Servings: 4

Ingredients:

Eggplants – 2

Black pepper, ground - .25 teaspoon

Extra virgin olive oil – 2 tablespoons

Cornstarch – 1 tablespoon

Basil, dried – 1 teaspoon

Garlic powder - .25 teaspoon

Sea salt - .5 teaspoon

Mayonnaise, made with olive oil - .5 cup

Garlic, minced – 1 teaspoon

Basil, fresh, chopped – 1 tablespoon

Lemon juice – 1 teaspoon

Chipotle, ground - .5 teaspoon

Sea salt - .25 teaspoon

Directions:

Begin by preheating your oven to Fahrenheit at four-hundred and twenty-five degrees. Place a wire cooking/cooling rack on a baking sheet.

Remove the peel from the eggplants and then slice them into rounds, each about three-quarters of an inch thick. Slice the rounds into wedges one inch in width.

Add the eggplant wedges to a large bowl and toss them with the olive oil. Once coated, add the pepper, cornstarch, dried basil, garlic powder, and sea salt, tossing until evenly coated.

Arrange the eggplant wedges on top of the wire rack and set the baking sheet in the oven, allowing the fries to cook for fifteen to twenty minutes.Meanwhile, prepare the aioli. To do this, add the remaining ingredients into a small bowl and whisk them together to combine. Cover the bowl of aioli and allow it to chill in the fridge until the fries are ready to be served.Remove the fries from the oven immediately upon baking, or allow them to cook under the broiler for an additional three to four minutes for extra crispy fries. Serve immediately with the aioli.

Nutrition:Energy (calories): 632 kcal Protein: 11.64 g Fat: 37.26 g Carbohydrates: 73.98 g

41. Eggplant Caponata

Preparation time: 10 minutes

Cooking time: 3minutes

Servings: 4

Time to Prepare/Cook: 25 minutes

Ingredients:

Eggplant, sliced into 1.5-inch cubes – 1 pound

Bell pepper, diced – 1

Green and black olives, chopped - .5 cup

Capers - .25 cup

Sea salt – 1 teaspoon

Garlic, minced – 4

Red onion, diced – 1

Diced tomatoes – 15 ounces

Extra virgin olive oil – 4 tablespoons, divided

Black pepper, ground - .25 teaspoon

Parsley, chopped - .25 cup

Directions:

Preheat your oven to Fahrenheit four-hundred degrees and line a baking sheet with kitchen parchment.

Toss the eggplant cubes in half of the olive oil and then arrange them on the baking sheet, sprinkling the sea salt over the top. Allow the eggplant to roast until tender, about twenty minutes.

Meanwhile, add the remaining olive oil into a large skillet and red onions, bell pepper, diced tomatoes, and garlic. Sauté the vegetables until tender, about ten minutes.

Add the roasted eggplant, capers, olives, and black pepper to the skillet, continuing to cook together for five minutes so that the flavors meld.

Remove the skillet from the heat, top it off with parsley, and serve it with crusty toast.

Nutrition: calories: 209

42. Buckwheat Crackers

Preparation time: 10 minutes

Cooking time: 60 minutes

Servings: 12

Ingredients:

Buckwheat groats – 2 cups

Flaxseeds, ground - .75 cup

Sesame seeds - .33 cup

Sweet potatoes, medium, grated – 2

Extra virgin olive oil – .33 cup

Water – 1 cup

Sea salt – 1 teaspoon

Directions:

Soak the buckwheat groats in water for at least four hours before preparing the crackers. Once done soaking, drain off the water.

Preheat the oven to a Fahrenheit temperature of three-hundred and fifty degrees, prepare a baking sheet, and set aside some kitchen parchment and plastic wrap.

In a kitchen bowl, combine the ground flaxseeds with the warm water, allowing the seeds to absorb the water and form a substance similar to gelatin. Add the buckwheat groats and other remaining ingredients.

Spread the cracker dough onto a sheet of kitchen parchment and cover it with a plastic wrap sheet. Use a rolling pin on top of the plastic wrap (so it doesn't stick) and roll out the buckwheat cracker dough until it is thin. Peel the plastic wrap off of the crackers and transfer the dough-coasted sheet of kitchen parchment to the prepared baking sheet. Allow it to partially bake for fifteen minutes and then remove the tray from the oven. Reduce the oven temperature to Fahrenheit three-hundred degrees. Use a pizza cutter and slice the crackers into squares, approximately two inches in width.

Return the crackers to the oven until they are crispy and dry, about thirty-five to forty minutes.

Remove the oven's crackers, allowing them to cool completely before storing them in an air-tight container.

Nutrition:

Energy (calories): 1087 kcal

Protein: 28.52 g Fat: 75.23 g

Carbohydrates: 88.41 g

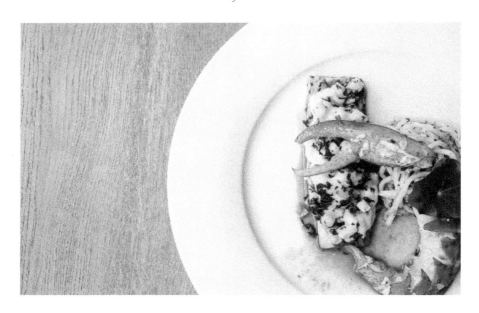

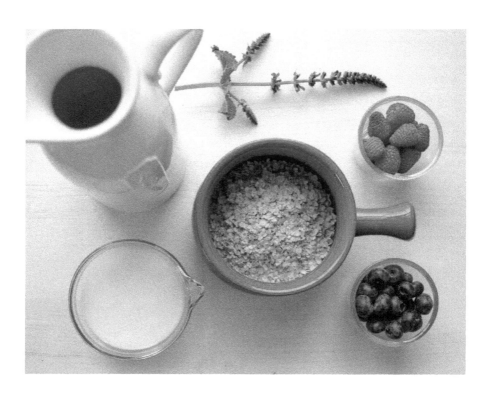

CHAPTER 15:

Desserts

43.   Cabbage Chips

Preparation Time: 10 minutes

Cooking time: 10 minutes

Servings: 2

Ingredients:

1cup of black cabbage

6 tbsp. of extra virgin olive oil

1 tbsp. of flax seeds

1 tbsp. of sesame seeds

Salt

Pepper

Directions:

First, clean the cabbage, then dry the leaves with a cloth and remove the central rib.

Prepare the dressing in a bowl by mixing salt, pepper, oil, and seeds.

Arrange the leaves on the baking tray lined with parchment paper without overlapping them, and then sprinkle them with the dressing.

Then cook for 5-10 minutes, or until they are crunchy, at 180 ° C in a preheated oven.

The black cabbage chips are ready, serve them immediately, whole or chopped.

Nutrition:

Calories: 4 Carbohydrate: 1g

Fat: 0 g Protein: 3 g

44. Savory Mushroom Muffins

Preparation Time: 10 minutes

Cooking time: 10 minutes

Servings: 8

Ingredients:

½ cup of 00 flour

2 tbsp. of parmesan

1/2 sachet of instant yeast for savory pies

1cup of milk

One egg

1 cup of mushrooms in oil

Salt

Pepper

Directions:

In a bowl, whisk the egg and milk, apart from mixing the flour, Parmesan and baking powder, salt, and pepper.

Add the flour and parmesan compote to the beaten egg and milk and mix everything with a wooden spoon.

Add mushroom in oil to dough, then lift them with a fork from a jar.

Stir quickly with a spoon so that the mushrooms are evenly distributed in the muffin dough

Pour the salted mushroom muffin mixture into buttered and floured muffin molds.

Turn on the oven at 180 degrees and cook for 20 minutes.

Leave to cool, and then serve your mushroom muffins.

Nutrition:

Calories: 182

Carbohydrate: 6g

Fat: 11 g

Protein: 10g

45.   Avocado Fries

Preparation Time: 10 minutes

Cooking time: 15 minutes

Servings: 4

Ingredients:

Two avocados

Three eggs

Rice flour

Breadcrumbs

1lime

Cumin

Pepper

Salt

Seed oil

Directions:

Cut the avocado in half and remove the core and cut it into sticks. Then remove the peel

Beat the eggs with the salt, pepper, cumin, and grated lime zest.

Pass the avocado sticks first in the flour, then in the eggs and breadcrumbs. Then again in the eggs and breadcrumbs, thus obtaining a double breading.

Fry the avocado sticks in hot oil. When they are golden brown, drain, and place the fries obtained on a plate covered with paper towels.

Serve the avocado sticks immediately, accompanying them with the mayonnaise you have flavored with juice and lime peel.

Nutrition:

Calories: 131.9

Carbohydrate: 6.6g

Fat: 11.1 g Protein: 4g

46.   Fruit Baskets

Preparation Time: 10 minutes

Cooking time: 20 minutes

Servings: 4

Ingredients

For the shortcrust pastry:

1cup of 00 flour

1egg

1cup of icing sugar

1 cup of butter

Lemon peel

For the cream:

Two yolks

5oz. of sugar

88oz. of 00 flour

9oz. of milk

Vanilla bean

Lemon peel

To garnish:

1/2 kiwi

4oz. of strawberries

3oz. of blueberries

Mint

Directions:

Start preparing the pastry by adding flour, eggs, sugar, grated lemon peel, and butter chunks. Work with your fingertips, starting from the center and gradually incorporating all the flour.

Once you have obtained homogeneous dough, wrap it in plastic wrap and leave it in the fridge for 30 minutes.

Once the dough is taken, roll it out on a floured work surface, obtaining a sheet of about 3mm.

With a pasta bowl, make circles and transfer them into the tart molds.

Prick the base with the prongs of a fork, and then cook the pastry shells in a preheated oven at 180 ° C for 15-20 minutes. Once ready, let it cool.

Now prepare the custard by adding the yolks and sugar.

Then add the flour and work until you get a cream.

Heat the milk with the vanilla stick and the lemon peel over the heat.

Before it reaches a boil, lift vanilla and lemon and transfer them to the prepared mixture.

Stir and pass everything on the fire to thicken.

Pour the cream into a bowl, cover with the cling film and allow cooling completely.

Clean the fruit and cut it into small pieces.

Now fill the baskets of pastry with the cream, using a syringe for sweets.

Finally, garnish with the pieces of fruit and mint leaves. Your fruit baskets are ready to be served.

Nutrition:

Calories: 100

Carbohydrate: 23g

Fat: 0 g Protein: 1g

47.   Mushroom And Tofu Scramble

Preparation time: 10 minutes

Cooking time: 20 minutes

Servings: 2

Ingredients

7 ounces of extra firm tofu

Two teaspoon turmeric powder

One teaspoon black pepper

1.5ounce of kale, roughly chopped

Two teaspoons extra virgin olive oil

1.5ounce of red onion, thinly sliced

1 Thai chili, thinly sliced

100g mushrooms, thinly sliced

Four tablespoons parsley, finely chopped

Directions

Wrap the tofu in paper towels and place something heavy on top to help it drain. Mix the turmeric with a little water until you achieve a light paste.

Steam the kale for 2 to 3 minutes.

Heat the olive oil in a frying pan over medium heat until hot but not smoking. Add the onion, chili, and mushrooms and fry for 2 to 3 minutes until they have started to brown and soften. Crumble the tofu into bite-size pieces, add to the pan, pour the turmeric paste over the tofu, and mix thoroughly. Add the black pepper and stir.

Cook over medium heat for 2 - 3 minutes so the spices are cooked through, and the tofu has started to brown.

Add the kale and continue to cook over medium heat for another minute. Finally, add the parsley, mix well, and serve.

Nutrition

Energy (calories): 663 kcal

Protein: 38.65 g

Fat: 26.54 g

Carbohydrates: 86.93 g

48.   Kale Scramble

Preparation time: 10 minutes

Cooking time: 6 minutes

Servings: 2

Ingredients

Four eggs

1/8 teaspoon ground turmeric

Salt and ground black pepper, to taste

One tablespoon water

Two teaspoons olive oil

1 cup fresh kale, tough ribs removed and chopped

Directions

In a bowl, add the eggs, turmeric, salt, black pepper, and water, and with a whisk, beat until foamy. In a wok, heat the oil over medium heat. Add the egg mixture and stir to combine. Immediately, reduce the heat to medium-low and cook for about 1–2 minutes, stirring frequently. Stir in the kale and cook for about 3–4 minutes, stirring frequently. Remove from the heat and serve immediately.

Nutrition   Energy (calories): 196 kcal Protein: 10.59 g Fat: 14.39 g Carbohydrates: 6.94 g

49.   Apple Pancakes With Blackcurrant Compote

Preparation time: 10 minutes

Cooking time: 20 minutes

Servings: 2

Ingredients

4 ounce of porridge oats

1.8ounce of plain flour

One tablespoon caster sugar

½ teaspoon baking powder

One large green apple, peeled, cored, and cut into small pieces

150ml semi-skimmed milk

I large egg white

One teaspoon light olive oil.

For the compote:

1.5ounce of blackcurrants washed and stalked removed.

One tablespoon caster sugar

Two tablespoon water.

Directions

Make the compote first. Place the blackcurrants, sugar, and water in a small pan. Bring to a simmer and cook for 10-15 minutes.

Place the Oats, flour, baking powder, and caster sugar in a large bowl and mix properly.

Stir the apple into the powder mixture and then whisk in the milk a little at a time until you have a smooth variety.

Whisk the egg white to a stiff peak and then fold into the pancake batter.

Heat ½ teaspoon olive oil in a non-stick frying pan on medium heat and pour ½ of the batter. Reduce heat and allow the pancake to cook correctly, flip to the other side with a spatula. Cook both sides until golden brown. Remove and repeat to make two pancakes.

Serve the pancakes with the blackcurrant compote drizzled over.

Nutrition

123 calories

50.　Mushroom Scramble Egg

Preparation Time: 5 minutes

Cooking time: 10 minutes

Servings: 3

Ingredients

Two eggs

One teaspoon ground turmeric

One teaspoon mild curry powder

20g kale, roughly chopped

One teaspoon extra virgin olive oil

½ bird's eye chili, thinly sliced

A handful of thinly sliced button mushrooms

5g parsley, finely chopped

Directions

Mix the curry and turmeric powder, then add a little water until a light paste has been achieved.

Steam up the kale for 2–3 minutes.

At medium heat, heat the oil in a frying pan and fry the chili and mushrooms for 2–3 minutes till they start browning and softening.

Put the eggs and spice paste, cook over medium heat, add the kale, and start cooking for another minute over medium heat. Add the parsley, then mix well and serve.

Nutrition

Energy (calories): 174 kcal

Protein: 10.57 g Fat: 12.16 g

Carbohydrates: 6.21 g

51. Sirtfood Mushroom Scramble Eggs

Preparation time: 10 minutes

Cooking time: 20 minutes

Servings: 1

Ingredients

Two medium eggs

I teaspoon turmeric

1 ounce of kale, roughly chopped

One teaspoon extra virgin olive oil

1/2 chili, thinly sliced

0.5 ounce of red onions

Parsley, thinly chopped

A handful of button mushrooms, thinly sliced

Directions

Steam the kale for 2-3 minutes.

Mix the turmeric powder with water to form a light paste.

Break into a bowl and whisk, add the turmeric paste, parsley, and mix properly.

Heat the olive oil in a non-stick frying pan over medium heat and fry the onion, chili, and mushroom until they have started to brown and soften.

Add the steamed kale to the mixture in the frying pan and stir.

Pour the egg mixture into the frying pan and stir.

Reduce the heat and allow the egg to cook and stir.

Nutrition:

Energy (calories): 131 kcal

Protein: 8.99 g

Fat: 6.95 g

Carbohydrates: 9.94 g

Conclusions

M ost diets have been proven to be just a temporary fix. If you want to keep weight off for a good while maintaining muscle mass and ensuring that your body stays healthy, then you need to be following a diet that activates your sirtuin genes: in other words, the Sirtfood Diet.

. But sirtuin genes aren't just responsible for weight loss and muscle gain—they also help prevent illnesses such as heart disease, diabetes, bone problems, Alzheimer's, and even cancer. To activate these genes, you must eat foods that are high in the plant-based proteins polyphenols. These are known as sirtfoods and include kale and walnuts and drinks such as green tea and red wine.

It is essential to eat a diet that combines whole, healthy, nutritious ingredients with various sirtfoods. These ingredients will all work together to increase the bioavailability of the sirtfoods even further. And there's no need to count calories: just focus on sensible portions and consume a diverse range of foods—including as many sirtfoods as you can and eating until you feel full.

You should also ensure you have a green sirtfood-rich juice every day to get all of those sirtuins- activating ingredients into your body. Also, feel free to indulge in tea, coffee, and the occasional glass of red wine. And most importantly, be adventurous. Now is the time to start leading a happy, healthy, and fat-free life without having to deprive you of delicious and satisfying food.